Fitness Knowledge

Beginner's Fitness Book

Written by:
Kym Stephens B.S., CFT and
Jay Walkins B.S., CFT

Kym Stephens holds a B.S. Degree in Exercise
Sciences and is a Certified Fitness Trainer

Jay Walkins holds a B.S. Degree in Exercise
Sciences, Nutrition and is a Certified Fitness Trainer

Jay Walkins is author of:
How to Be Healthy and Live Longer
(Know Health, Be Healthy and Live Longer)

And
How to Start a Running Routine and Become a Confident
Runner (A Beginner's Guide to Running and Jogging)

special or otherwise that may result from the information presented in this publication.

We have relied on my own experience as well as many different sources for this book, and we have done my best to check facts and to give credit where it is due.

Front Image: FreeDigitalPhotos.net

Table of Contents

Introduction

In 400 B.C. Hippocrates wrote the following: "Eating alone will not keep a man well; he must also take exercise. For food and exercise, while possessing opposite qualities, yet work together to produce health….And it is necessary, as it appears, to discern the power of various exercises, both natural exercises and artificial, to know which of them tends to increase flesh and which to lessen it; and not only this, but also to proportion exercise to bulk of food, to the constitution of the patient, to the age of the individual…"

From the beginning of recorded time, philosophers such as Hippocrates have observed that regular physical activity is an essential part of life. The Dead Sea scrolls (part of the Bible), one of the oldest written pieces of history, is filled with examples and reasons why a person's body must be in good health. Out of dozens of verses that discuss keeping the body healthy, one immediately comes to my mind; *"Or do you not know that your body is a temple of the Holy Spirit within you, whom you have from God? You are not your own, for you were bought with a price. So glorify God in your body."* 1 Corinthians 6:19-20.

So this is what I take from this verse: God is telling me to keep my body optimized, healthy and fit; to keep my body from impurities such has fatty foods, empty carbohydrates, smoking, alcohol and drugs, for God resides in my physical flesh; it is His temple!

In this book we will give you our *Fitness Knowledge*, but because there is so much to share with you, we can not possibly fit all that we know into a single book. Please look for other volumes and books written or brought to you by Jay Walkins or Kym Stephens!

Fitness 101

Based on their studies, the American College of Sports Medicine (ACSM), the Center for Disease Control (CDC) and the President's Council on Physical Fitness issued statements proclaiming that sedentary people can greatly reduce their risk of developing heart disease and other health problems by performing just thirty minutes of light to moderate activity 4 or more days of a week. Additional fitness benefits can result from going beyond that by increasing the frequency to three to five days per week of vigorous aerobic exercise. The greatest boost in improving the overall health of people comes from sedentary individuals beginning to do just a little bit of exercise every day!

Studies have shown active lifestyle enhances quality of life for individuals. An increase in total physical activity at low to moderate intensities is associated with a decrease in the risk of heart disease. Regular vigorous activity increases cardiorespiratory fitness.

Many people have used the term wellness to emphasize that positive health is much more than simply being free from illness; there is an additional quality to maintaining a health well-being. I use the term fitness to try and capture this same concept. Fitness is a condition reached through striving for optimal quality of life in all aspects: social, mental, psychological, spiritual and physical. These aspects of fitness are interrelated; a high level in one of the areas enhances other areas, and, conversely, a low level in any area restricts the accomplishments possible in other areas. Physical activity can also contribute to learning ability and forming relationships.

Fitness and health can also be defined as being alive with no major health problems.
The primary health goals are to avoid premature death, or to delay death by avoiding a preventable disease.
However, the components related to these goals include heredity, environment, habits and general health status. Actions and behaviors that contribute to a healthy life are regular exercise, nutrition, adequate sleep, no tobacco use, no excess alcohol use and of course avoiding the use of non-essential drugs.

Ok, let's go over the physical and psychological benefits to being fit; we will start with the physical aspect. Your bones comes first to my mind, staying fit will actually help build bone mass. By building this bone mass and density, you will reduce your chances of developing osteoporosis, osteoarthritis and lower back pain. Being fit will reduce risk of heart disease, stroke and other vascular problems. I discuss this in further detail later in this book.

Staying fit will help burn calories and lower your risk of being overweight, or developing diabetes. Belly fat alone can produce inflammatory molecules thus leading to type two diabetes and heart disease. Time to get rid of that belly fat!

Another physical benefit is that being fit improves the function of your immune system.

A psychological benefit to being fit is that it will lower anxiety and or depression. There have been studies that found exercise as effective as psychotherapy in reducing depression.

Exercise and being fit will control stress and minimize its effects on the body.
Fitness will give you self-esteem and this will improve how you feel and what you think about yourself. A fit person's mind tends to correlate with improved cognition and problem solving skills.
Keep in mind that our bodies were designed to be active and moving; not just sitting around watching the television.

Fitness is divided into two parts: aerobic fitness and muscular fitness.
Aerobic fitness is your ability to carry out continuous activities such as walking, running, cycling, cross country skiing and other actions that require large muscle activities.
When you engage in these types of activities at a level above your normal daily level, you overload your muscles including your heart and lungs. If you repeat this regularly, say every other day, your body will begin to adapt to this overload by the exercise. As you improve

your aerobic fitness, you are also enhancing the ability to burn fat.
Muscular fitness includes strength, muscle endurance and flexibility.

Here is an interesting fact: as you become fit, particularly with aerobic fitness training, your blood volume will increase and your heart will pump more blood throughout your body.

Your Heart Is an Engine

Your heart is the little engine that keeps your body and assembly line going. It takes oxygenated blood from the lungs and pumps it throughout the whole body, and then the heart takes carbon dioxide in the blood back from the body and pumps it into the lungs where it is exchanged for more oxygen.

Your heart began pumping before you were born and it will continue pumping until the day you die. A well-conditioned and fit man who exercises regularly will have a resting heart rate of approximately sixty beats per minute or less. A deconditioned man who does not exercise regularly will have a sitting heart rate of eighty beats or more.

Women have slightly higher heart rates than men, as do children. Obesity, stress and other factors can speed the heart rate up, even though a person may appear to be in good condition.

Suppose that a person were at a complete rest for a full twenty four hours, a comparison might go something like this:

A. Sixty beats per minute, times sixty minutes equals 3,600 beats per hour, times 24 hours equals 86,400 bets per day.

B. Eighty beats per minute, times sixty minutes equals 4,800 beats per hour, times 24 hours equals 115,200 beats per day.

A deconditioned man at complete rest who does not exercise his heart, forces to pump nearly 30,000 more times during everyday of his life!

The heart is all muscle and has three different sizes: a normal but deconditioned heart is relatively small and weak due to lack of proper exercise. This type of heart will eventually atrophy and waste away. The second type is an enlarged unhealthy heart that normally grows to compensate for a deficiency in the cardiovascular system. The interior of this enlarged heart, despite their exterior size, is not as large so they cannot pump as much blood with each stroke. Lastly, an athlete's heart is strong and healthy and is relatively large, pumping more blood with less effort for each stroke.

Conditioned hearts as they grow larger and stronger may beat more slowly because they're pumping more blood with each stroke. Nearly all great distance runners have low heart rates. Some runners are reported to have a resting heart rate of 32 beats per minute compared to a young office worker that has a heart rate of about 75 to 80.

To determine your heart rate at rest, sit still for five minutes in front of a clock then take your pulse and count the beats for a full sixty seconds. If your heart rate is eighty beats or above you are not in good condition. The first thing you need to do is start being more active.

A well-conditioned heart also reduces the maximum heart rates, which is just as important as resting heart rates. Healthy hearts will peak, without strain, at approximately 190 beats per minute or less, while unconditioned hearts may go as high as 220 beats per minute. Unconditioned hearts that beat this rapidly creates a dangerous health situation.

There is another heart rate that has nothing to do with physical exercise. It is called the anticipatory rate. You can think of it as an emotional heart rate. A balloon pops unexpectedly near you and you can feel your heart rate instantly pound and race. Your boss calls you into his office to scold you, and you can feel your heart race faster. All of these little scares have a cumulative effect on the heart; a conditioned heart can reduce this effect.

Heart Disease and Cardiovascular Problems

Cardiovascular problems cause the majority of premature deaths in the U.S., and those that survive these problems have severe limitations in their lives. There are many different forms of these heart problems. Here is the run down.

1) *Arteriosclerosis* is an arterial disease, hardening and thickening of vessel walls.

2) *Atherosclerosis* is fatty substances that are deposited in the inner walls of the arteries.

3) *Coronary Artery Thrombosis* is occlusion of a coronary artery by a blood clot.

4) *Coronary Heart Disease (CHD)* is atherosclerosis of the coronary arteries, also called coronary artery disease (CAD).

5) *Embolism* is a sudden obstruction of a blood vessel by a solid body such as a clot carried in the blood stream.

6) *Heart Attack* a term used to describe an acute episode of heart disease; common name for myocardial infarction.

7) *Hypertension* is high blood pressure. When you take your blood pressure, there is a top number and a bottom number, systolic is the top and diastolic is the bottom. If the bottom diastolic number exceeds 90, then the person

being tested is considered to be suffering from hypertension.

8) Myocardial Infarction (MI) is death to a section of the heart tissue in which the blood supply has been cut off.

9) **Thrombosis** is a blood clot in a blood vessel.

10) **Cholesterol** is fatty substance in which carbon, hydrogen and oxygen atoms are arranged in rings.

CHD is the leading cause of premature death in the U.S. and cholesterol is predominant in the plaque that clogs up the arteries. High blood pressure (hypertension) is the most common cardiovascular disease. Hypertension is related to CHD and stroke. Stroke is the result of obstructions or hemorrhages of blood vessels in the brain. It usually results in an abrupt disruption of bodily function and loss of consciousness and may cause partial paralysis. There is some evidence that regular exercise reduces the risk of stroke.

Sedentary people should work towards performing at least thirty minutes of daily moderate exercise to reduce their risk of heart disease. See Aerobic Fitness section for further explanation.

High Blood Pressure and Factors Involved

In about ninety to ninety five percent of cases, the cause of high blood pressure is unknown. Although the specific cause isn't known, there are contributing factors involved.

Let's start with the uncontrollable factors. The first and foremost uncontrollable factors are age, race, heredity and sex. The older a person gets, the more likely he or she is to develop high blood pressure. African Americans have high blood pressure more often than Caucasians. It also tends to occur earlier and be more severe in African Americans.
A tendency toward high blood pressure seems to run in families as well. Men are more likely to develop high blood pressure than women, but this varies by age and among ethnic groups.

There are five controllable factors right off the top: obesity, sodium intake, alcohol consumption, oral contraceptives and physical inactivity.
Obesity is being thirty percent or more over ideal body weight. Obesity and blood pressure are clearly related. That's why all obese hypertensive adults should try to get within fifteen percent of their desirable body weight.

Reducing sodium (salt) consumption can lower blood pressure in some people.
Drinking more than one ounce of alcohol a day may increase blood pressure in some people.
Women who take oral contraceptives may develop high blood pressure.
Lack of exercise, physical activity and living a sedentary life style contributes to obesity.

As many as ninety million Americans aged sixty and above have high blood pressure.
Besides claiming lives, high blood pressure is also indirectly responsible for deaths and disability resulting from heart attack, stroke and kidney failure. According to estimates by the American Heart Association, one in four Americans aged eighteen and over have high blood pressure.

Lastly to recap, the most common treatments for high blood pressure are reducing salt intake, losing weight and exercising more often.

Aerobic Fitness

Aerobic fitness can be improved by training at an intensity level just above light effort but below hard exertion. For many years people believed that raising the heart rate was a good gauge to measure intensity; this is not true. If you engage large muscle mass in activity (muscle mass is fueled by oxidation of fat and carbohydrates), you will achieve the desired level of intensity without overworking the heart.

Intensity and duration work hand in hand; if you increase one, then you must decrease the other out of necessity. Three factors that are related with duration are, time, distance and calories used. Speaking of calories, food and beverage labels give a good idea how many calories you consume. For example, one beer will supply about one hundred calories; this info on the label can be used to find the specific exercise that will be needed to balance your energy intake. Here is an example of what I'm saying: a good run on the treadmill for one mile will use a little more than hundred calories, so to burn that hundred calorie beer off, and you would need to jog on that treadmill just under a mile.
Before you eat and drink, think of what you must do to balance your energy intake and energy output.

A unit of energy is known as a calorie. A calorie is the amount of heat required to raise the temperature of one liter of water by one degree Celsius. Calories are stored when you eat, and burned away when you exercise; the rate at which they are burned is influenced by how much you weigh.
A lighter person will burn fewer calories than a heavier person while running at the same pace.

In this book, calorie output is based on the weight of a150 pound person. If you are not at 150 pounds, you can adjust the numbers by adding or subtracting ten percent for every fifteen pounds over or under 150. When a person at 150 pounds is running, they will lose about 113 calories per mile. If you weigh 165 lbs. then add ten percent to the 113 calories in order to find how many calories you would burn while running a mile (113x0.10=11.3+113= 124.3 calories).

By taking on three training sessions per week on alternating days, a sedentary person can increase their aerobic fitness. By increasing their frequency of training, the unfit individual will improve their fitness in intensity and duration as their training progresses.

An over weight person will need to exercise more frequently if they want to have better weight control. Exercising five days versus two days a week will have a much better effect achieving good fitness and weight loss. It's also critical to keep in mind to never over train the body.

Over training can cause many bad effects on the body, such as injury and illness by suppressing your immune system. The body needs to recover fully from training sessions or you won't get the most out of your fitness program.

To give your body time to rest and recover, you must progress gradually so that your body can adjust to the training. The unfit person living a sedentary life must become active before implementing training; an example of an activity would be a brisk walk. After your body has adapted to this activity, you may begin Aerobic Fitness as a beginner with a training exercise, such as running, jogging, cycling, paddling, swimming, etc.

The frequency for training of a beginner would be two to four days a week; the frequency for a person with an intermediate level of fitness would be five to six while advanced would be six or more days per week.

Muscular Fitness

Firefighters and construction workers are just a few examples of professionals that use muscular fitness day to day. However, a person that's not in this type of field can surely benefit as well by developing muscular fitness. An overweight person can burn away fat by developing muscular strength; as muscle mass increases it will eat and burn fat.

You can avoid any future problems with osteoporosis (loss of bone density) by doing load bearing muscular activities and exercises. Examples of load bearing exercise would be squats, leg presses, shoulder press, free weights, machines and many more.

There are many factors involved with muscular fitness such as coordination, agility, power, and the three top ones are muscular endurance, strength and flexibility. As we grow older, these attributes with muscular fitness will decline and disappear.
This rate of decline can be significantly reduced by being active and maintaining a regimen that focuses on muscular fitness.

I have had clients in their ninety's who has developed muscular strength and muscle mass. The human body can not be slowed down if the correct steps are taken consistently.

Here is a true story. I had a client from 2006-2007 name Charlie and he was 93 years old. Charlie lived two homes down from me. He became aware that I was a fitness trainer and asked if he could work with me. I had a home gym and twice a week Charlie would come over for 30 minutes for muscular fitness training. In the beginning his arms were flabby with no tone, and he had inches around his waist line. Charlie couldn't even pick up a 3 lbs dumbbell.
Within three weeks Charlie was lifting 25 lbs. dumbbells and his arm had hardened like a rock. His flabby arms had literally melted away.

If older people do not take up muscular activities and exercises, they will continue through a process known as Sarcopenia a.k.a. vanishing of the flesh. This is why they have higher rates of falls and fractures; the loss of muscle fibers is from the lack of use.

Let's look at the factors again involved with muscular fitness starting with muscular strength:
Lifting heavy loads creates strength. Strength is the maximal force that a person can exert in a single voluntary contraction. This amount of force is called 1 repetition maximum.

In order to minimize injuries and to handle emergencies, muscular strength is needed at a moments notice. Muscular strength is used every time you pick up the grocery bags or take out the trash.

The difference between muscular strength and muscular endurance is that muscular strength is needed only when want to lift a heavy box one time. Muscular endurance is needed when that heavy box needs to be lifted many times.

To repeat muscular contractions for a period of time, muscular endurance is going to be needed. Examples would be loading a moving truck, or walking a golfing course.

Contracting muscle fibers repeatedly will achieve muscular endurance. You enhance the aerobic enzymes within the muscles that helps feed them by doing repetitive contractions such as bicycling or a stationary bicycle.

Aerobic endurance and muscular endurance are two different things. A guitar player, or say a massage therapist, will develop endurance in the finger muscles but this will not have an effect on his or her heart. A massage therapist may have great endurance in the hands but his or her aerobic fitness may be horrible.

Flexibility

Limbs move in a range of motion called flexibility. Your skin, connective tissue and joints can limit your range of motion. In addition, body fat also can limit your range of motion and flexibility. Injuries can occur if you force a limb beyond its normal flexibility range. However, injury can be reduced as your flexibility improves. Stretching also contributes to increased range of motion.

An important fact to remember is that your body must be warmed up prior to stretching cold muscles. An example of a warm up would be a fast-paced walk on the treadmill for approximately 10 minutes.

If you have been to a gym, you have probably noticed most people stretching their muscles incorrectly. You probably have witnessed those individuals stretching cold muscles before completing their warm up. This is a big mistake! Additionally, as one gets older, stretching becomes an important factor in keeping range of motion at its greatest. Seniors can benefit from regular stretching as their connective tissue becomes less elastic as they progress in age.

Speed and Power

Fast twitch muscle fibers provide rapid acceleration, also known as speed. The combination of speed and strength equals power, also known as force. An example of the need for power would be in a game of football where explosive force comes from the lineman's leg, arm, chest and back muscles to move his opponent backwards. In fact, just about all sports require power and speed.

To increase your power for use in a certain sport or activity, be sure remember the principle of specificity. For example, if you are a runner you can increase your running power by lifting weights, running uphill and running against resistance.

Balance

Balance can be dynamic or it can be static. To keep your balance while you are not moving is the definition of static balance. Static balance is crucial in many activities such as mountain biking, keeping your balance on a ladder or mountain climbing. The ability to maintain equilibrium while you are in motion defines dynamic balance. You are using this dynamic balance during simple activities such as walking around, walking up and down the stairs and playing sports. Most people demonstrate good dynamic balance and poor static balance. Both static and dynamic balance contributes to performance in sports and regular activities on a daily basis. A person can improve their balance by participating in activities such as Yoga, Tai Chi, Chi Gung and other related activities.

Agility

An individual that can change direction precisely and rapidly, without losing their balance, has good agility. Agility encompasses and depends upon speed, strength, coordination and balance. Excessive weight training can hinder your agility. Muscular endurance along with aerobic endurance will help you maintain agility for long periods.

Coordination

Movement with a smooth flow as tasks are executed is known as coordination.
When executing a tennis serve, for example, force is created through a series of movements. Momentum first develops from turning your body, and then at the height of that momentum, your arm extends at the elbow,

followed by a burst of your maximum possible racket speed brought on by the snap of the wrist.

While some coordination may be inherited, skill is commonly achieved through regular practice. Keep in mind that if a skill is practiced incorrectly, bad habits that are hard to break will develop. It is critical to make sure you are practicing properly. When in doubt, look to a professional instructor in that particular field.

Shaping

The term 'getting in shape' is often tossed around. To achieve this goal, there are four steps to follow. They include losing excess weight which requires that you take in fewer calories than calories that are burned. This is accomplished through heightened aerobic activity such as running or swimming. The compliment to this step (losing excess weight) is taking in fewer foods that are highly-dense in calories such as desserts, dressings, or large fatty meals that cause you to feel overly full rather than eating small meals throughout the day.

The next step is to improve your muscle tone. To curb boredom with your program and to improve muscle tone, vary your activities and add strength training with weights. Additionally, make core training and flexibility a part of the program.

Posture is the third component. As you are losing excess weight and increasing strength, realize that posture is not to be overlooked. Standing tall with your shoulders back and head forward makes you not only feel better but you will also look better. Make core exercises a part of your routine to improve posture.

The final component is increasing the size of your muscles. The term hypertrophy is defined as an increase to the mass of muscle by an increase in the individual fibers of the muscle. This can be accomplished through strength training. An example of this is performing 10 to 15 repetitions at your maximum weight. Thus, for 10 to 15 repetitions you lift the maximum weight you are able to lift.

When executing the above goals, you may want to consult with various fitness tables to evaluate where you stand in obtaining your goal. At whatever point in your program, you may desire to do a fitness test to see where you stand. As you progress, you can re-evaluate and thus determine what needs improvement.

Principle of Overload

What is overload? Research shows that in order to increase or improve, you need to overload or place demand on the body systems. How much should you overload? In order to improve strength, one needs to overload or inflict a demand that is greater than two-thirds of the maximal force of the muscle. This load or demand will need to be continually increased; the amount to increase is determined by intensity, duration and how often you train.

Since we are all at various levels, keep these pointers in mind. For instance, if you are new to strength training, try light weights and resistance bands. Work your way slowly from there. At the intermediate level, you are progressing so you will need greater resistance to keep improving. Try weight machines and calisthenics as they do not require the same amount of supervision as free weights. Finally, for the advanced levels, work with free weights and strength machines as they are more multipurpose. You will want to rely on a spotter (someone who makes sure a barbell won't fall on you while bench-pressing, or that you are able to make it up for your final repetition of a weighted-squat) for those moments when safety is in jeopardy.

Muscle Soreness

Muscle soreness is an often unwelcome friend when training. You will probably experience this in the beginning as your muscles are becoming used to being worked to their capacity. Keep working the program as the soreness will taper. As you continue your program, you may experience muscle soreness from overdoing your training. This often occurs 24 hours later and is referred to as DOMS or delayed-onset muscle soreness.

There are many possible causes to DOMS such as small tears in the connective tissue, damage to the muscle fiber, swelling or excess fluid called edema, contractions of the muscle fibers that are uncontrollable or even the effects of metabolic by-products hanging around in your muscles. While you may be thinking the soreness is solely caused by lactic acid, research actually shows that by-product escapes from your system within an hour following your workout.

As you start an exercise program, progress gradually from light weights to heavier weights (when you are ready). Also, practice patience by stretching your muscles before and after an activity; it is worth the time that it takes. Additionally, your body will require time to adapt to a new program when involving new ballistic or high energy movements.

Increasing Muscular Endurance and Strength

Remember that increases in strength do not happen overnight, but gradually. The key is to keep at the program; consistency is key! In general, you should see a 1 to 3 percent increase in your strength for each week. If you are new to strength training, your results will happen faster and will plateau as you reach your potential maximum strength. Over the course of 6 months, you can attain an increase in strength of 50 percent or more.

Tips to Keep In Mind When Training

- Choose 8 to 10 exercises that coincide with your training goals.

- Start off easy with sets that are lighter. A good rule of thumb is to do a 15 to 25 repetition maximum and work towards an increased load of a 10 repetition maximum.

- Breathing is very important. You will want to exhale on the exertion, or when you lift a weight and inhale on the lowering of the weight. Think of blowing the weight up ("blow out the candles") and inhale ("smell the flowers") as you lower. You may be tempted to hold your breath especially during difficult lifts. Avoid this habit as holding your breath can increase your blood pressure to a dangerous level and cause your heart to work much harder. The blood that is returned to your heart and the flow of blood circulating in your coronary arteries can be severely restricted simply by holding your breath; you heart will be lacking oxygen. In addition to the aforementioned, several episodes of breath-holding can lead to a hernia from the intra-abdominal pressure.

- Bring a friend for those lifts where you need a spotter. Safety is key!

- When completing sets for strength, allow your body 2 to 3 minutes of rest between the sets for the same exercise. Give yourself 1 to 2 minutes for muscular endurance training.

- Start off with two sessions of training per week for the first several weeks. From there, increase to three sessions per week.

- Give yourself 48 hours between working the same muscles. One way to accomplish this is to workout every other day such as Monday, Wednesday and Friday.

- Keep good notes of your progress. This can include your maximum strength, body weight and even measurements of dimensions that are important to you (i.e. chest, biceps, waist, etc.).

Nutrition

Whether you are implementing or enhancing an exercise program, the fuel from nutrition is definitely a key player. You will need sufficient energy, specifically protein, carbohydrates and healthy fats. As you consume and digest food, it is absorbed into the bloodstream as fuel and is circulated throughout your body. The enzymes found in the metabolic pathways then convert into other high energy substances to fuel the muscles.

Every person expends energy whether they are moving or not. In fact, a person weighing approximately 150 pounds and lying in bed for 24 hours would still burn nearly 1600 calories. That would be enough to power organs like the heart and lungs, control cellular metabolism and regulate body temperature. Mental activity such as deep-thinking only slightly increases energy expenditure, however, simply moving around increases your output of energy dramatically. When it comes down to it, activity that is physical in nature has the most dramatic effect on energy needs.

Carbohydrate

For this fuel, there are two kinds, simple and complex. The simple kind is a simple sugar. It offers some energy, but is limited in some nutrients like vitamins and minerals. Included in this category are glucose, fructose and sucrose.

The complex carbohydrate is crucial to your body's performance as it offers nutrients and fiber. Some foods of this nature are beans, brown rice and whole grain products like bread or pasta. Remember half of your daily calories should come from complex carbohydrates.

Comparing a performance diet to an average diet would include different composite percentages. An average diets percentage of daily calories would be around 45 to 50 percent from carbohydrates, 35 to 40 percent from fat and 10 to 15 percent from protein. A performance diet would include 55 to 60 percent from carbohydrates, 25 to 30 percent from fat and 15 percent from protein.

Glycemic Index

The glycemic index is defined by the speed at which carbohydrate digestion affects the glucose levels in your blood. A high glycemic food is quickly digested and causes a rapid increase in the blood sugar whereas low glycemic foods are slower to digest and be absorbed.

This is due to the fiber and fat content in the low glycemic foods.

Let's compare some high, moderate or middle and low glycemic foods. Examples of high glycemic would include white bread, cereal (ones that do not have bran but do have high fructose corn syrup), sugar, baked potatoes and honey. The next level of moderate includes whole-grain breads, oatmeal, peas, bran, pasta and corn. Finally, the low glycemic level includes yogurt, an assortment of fruits, lentils, milk and beans.

The Process

After consuming a meal, your blood utilizes the sugars and circulates them to the areas in your body in this order: heart, skeletal muscle and liver. The heart requires this for energy as it is in constant motion. Skeletal muscles can store it away and use it at a later time. These granules of stored energy are called muscle glycogen. The liver also stores glucose, like the skeletal muscles, and it is also called glycogen. When there are excess stores of carbohydrate, the body naturally conserves it as fat.

Sometimes, during the circulation of blood glucose, there is not enough present in your system and you experience hypoglycemia. This is apparent through symptoms of confusion, cold sweat, vertigo, drowsiness, headaches, fatigue or exhaustion, irritability and even vision that is blurred.

Fat

Despite what you might believe, fat is still necessary to the body. It is responsible for making up the membranes of your cells and the insulation throughout your nervous system. In addition, it is important to the compounds like hormones and as a shock absorber for the body's internal organs. During long bouts of sustained energy or endurance, fat is necessary as a form of fuel. A typical day, however, should only include 25 percent of the daily calories from fat with 33 percent or lower from fats that are saturated.

Protein

Protein serves an important role in the active lifestyle. Whether you eat animal or plant proteins, amino acids are created from the breakdown of its large molecules. They are utilized in the building of cell membranes, muscle tissue, enzymes, hormones and many other molecules. Protein is not a major contributor to energy during rest or exercise. Conversely, if you do heavy exercise during the process of dieting to lose weight, the body can go into starvation mode. Sensing this by the body will cause the protein of tissue to be used as a source of energy. This means you will lose muscle tissue. Allow yourself to stick to a 15 percent ratio of protein coming from quality sources such as nuts, skinned poultry, meat that is lean, fish and beans.

You may question what would qualify as a serving of protein. Envision your protein source to a deck of cards. When it is cooked, it will be 2 to 3 ounces.

Vitamins

Throughout the previous reading, we have discussed fats, proteins and carbohydrates. They are also classified as macronutrients. Conversely, vitamins and minerals are called micronutrients due to the fact we only need a small amount in our daily diet. Despite this, they are still essential to cell metabolism, immunity, blood clotting ability and other roles.

Why are these micronutrients essential to the diet? The answer is their role with enzymes. Vitamins are considered coenzymes and they are the active part of the enzyme which executes life-essential tasks in the body's chemical reactions. In a typical day, eating a well-balanced diet provides vitamins and minerals that are required by the body. Supplementing with excess doses will not cause your body to work more efficiently, and in some cases, can even be toxic.

Vitamins have varying levels of solubility in fat or water. Water soluble vitamins are of the B complex and vitamin C. When these are taken in high doses, they are washed out of the body through urine. While it is difficult to build up a toxic amount of water-soluble vitamins, it is easy to have a deficiency. On the other side of the spectrum are the fat-soluble vitamins which are found when you ingest fat. These include vitamins A, D, E and K. When these fat-soluble vitamins are in excess, they are not flushed out of the body but are stored away in the tissue of the body. Unless you are following a fat-restrictive diet, you generally will not have a deficiency of these types of vitamins.

The Effect of Vitamins on Immunity

When choosing what foods you want to include in your diet, you will want to remember these vital micronutrients found in these foods.

- Beta Carotene helps the cells of your immune system fight infection. It is found in sweet potatoes and carrots.

- Vitamin B_6 helps to make white blood cells. Some sources of this vitamin are spinach, potatoes and nuts.

- Folate increases the activity of white blood cells and is found in salmon, peas and romaine lettuce.

- Vitamin C is an antioxidant and is responsible for improving immunity response. Citrus fruits, peppers and broccoli are great sources of Vitamin C.

- Vitamin E is also an antioxidant that promotes immune response and is found in vegetable oils, whole grains and wheat germ.

Antioxidants

When you exercise at an intense level, free radical compounds are produced. These are harmful to the body and can even hurt your body's muscle tissue. To combat this, the body uses antioxidants which are found in limited supply in the body.

Antioxidants can be found in various food sources, and thus should be included in your diet. Keep in mind that antioxidants found in fruits and vegetables are far superior to antioxidants that are coming from vitamin supplements. In fact, there is a scale that lists the antioxidants found in foods, per 100 grams. It is called the ORAC scale (Oxygen Radical Absorbance Capacity). Just to name a few at the top of the chart, or best sources, are ground cloves, ground cinnamon, cocoa powder which is dry and unsweetened, dark chocolate and pecans.

Minerals

Minerals, like vitamins, are crucial to your body as they assist in enzyme and cellular activity, making of hormones, health of your bones, activity of muscles and nerves and the balance of acids and bases in your body. Minerals can be found in many dietary sources, although animal tissue and animal products provide higher amounts. If you take in a well-balanced diet on a regular basis, your body should be receiving appropriate amounts of nutrients. If you cut out a major source of nutrients, such as meat, this can have a harmful effect on your system.

Just like vitamins, minerals in excess can also cause harm like diarrhea (excess of magnesium or zinc), cirrhosis (excess of iron) and high blood pressure (excess of sodium). If you feel unsure of what the recommended dietary guidelines are, feel free to consult the U.S. Department of Health and Human Services at www.health.gov/dietaryguidelines.

Dispelling the Myths

There is an abundance of information out there today regarding fitness and nutrition. Some of it is true and much of it is false or misleading. Please read below for some of the common myths.

- Can muscle turn to fat and can fat turn into muscle? A fat cell and a muscle cell are not interchangeable. Each type of cell has a specific role in the body. Muscle cells are produced to exert force whereas fat cells are created to store fat.

- No pain, no gain! When you exercise, it is not required to reach a level of pain. Reaching a maximum repetition which causes you to need rest between sets is important. During the exercise or lift, for example, you may feel a burn sensation. This is usually from the buildup of lactic acid, which eventually goes away. Remember, lactic acid buildup is gone within an hour of your workout. If you are experiencing real pain while working out, you need to back off. Your body is giving you a warning.

- If I purchase that equipment from television, I will look just like the beautiful model showcasing it! Sticking to a consistent workout regimen and well-balanced diet will always reign superior to a beautiful, probably highly paid model or actor advertising the newest get-fit gimmick.

In the Long Run

Research has been conducted and studied regarding the relationship of health to an assortment of habits and behaviors. Improving your health and increasing the length of your life has been determined as directly proportional to the following…

- Eating a healthy breakfast

- Getting approximately 7 to 8 hours of sleep each night

- Consuming small meals throughout the day (approximately 4 meals)

- No smoking

- Controlling your weight

- Little to no alcohol

- A regular exercise routine

It was determined by the Human Population Laboratory that women could add seven years to their lives and men could add eleven years to their lives simply by adhering to six of these habits (Breslow and Enstrom 1980).

When looking into your own life to determine what habits you can include, remember it is about adding life to your years and not just years to your life.

- Moderation is important in all aspects whether it is exercise, work, diet or even pleasure.

- Flexibility is another characteristic, whether in the physical sense or psychological. One needs to be able to adapt and accept change.

- Give yourself a healthy dose of stress or challenge. If you do not have any, create some. If life becomes too challenging, allow yourself to recognize this and ask for help.

- Be a creature of healthy habits with everything in balance and moderation.

- Take a second look at the relationships in your life and value them. Older individuals tend to take stock and value their marriage and relationships with friends and family.

- Look at the glass as half full whenever you can. In doing so, you can accept and adapt to every stage of life that you are in. Be able to enjoy life!

- Keep an active lifestyle which in return offers you purpose and direction. This lifestyle should be active socially and physically.